Calisthenics Training For Beginners:

Calisthenics and Bodyweight Training, Workout, Exercise Guide

By

Charles Maldonado

Table of Contents

Calisthenics Training For Beginners: Calisthenics and Bodyweight Training, Workout, Exercise Guide

By Charles Maldonado

First Published, 2015

Printed in the United States of America

Introduction

Physical fitness and keeping a good body is no longer an option. To survive the toils of the modern world, you have to be fit and strong. This is why people visit the gym every now and then. At the gym, you will have the tools you need to work out and stay fit. What if there were no gyms. No weights or treadmills. How will you survive? Choosing an elaborate calisthenics workout schedule will ensure that you keep your body working optimally regardless of what you have around you.

While most of the calisthenics workout routines will focus on building your physique and inner strength without using any weights, paying attention to creativity and improvisation is the only way to ensuring that you get something that works for you. A perfect balance between complexity of a procedure and there alignment of your body as you do the reps will determine the target muscles and the benefits you reap off the workout routine. Using your body as the weight is good enough to ensure that you get the right physique and resilience. However, since most of the workout routines might push you to the limits, knowing a couple of the safety rules and safe procedures to follow should keep you safe throughout the workout sessions.

Chapter 1. Basic Principles of Calisthenics Training

Thanks to calisthenics, you can now get to work out on your fitness, physique, and body strength without the use of weights and machines. It is the art where you use your body weight and qualities of inertia. It was first developed by the Greeks many years back before mass gaining pills and the likes became a reality. It somehow beats logic to see people all over the world celebrate it like it was just invented the other day. Well, it may be a new phenomenon in some parts of the world thanks to the internet. It has also been documented which means that it now has a by-the-book procedure. Whatever the case, calisthenics is very effective. Considering the fact that very few people can acquire their own gym machinery or pay for gym membership, calisthenics happens to be a viable option.

The one good thing about calisthenics is that it involves the whole body during workouts. You actually get to work up the entire system cohesively. Some calisthenics exercises may put emphasis on specific body parts but it usually involves most parts of the body. For example, when doing one hand push-ups, you will need the strength and tension from the entire body. The strength of your arm alone will not be enough. It is a full-body work out.

The basic principle for any weight training exercise is progressive overload. With that being said, in calisthenics, we have three basic weight training exercises. They include; push-ups, pull-ups, and squats. From these three, you will get many different variations or innovations to serve varying purposes.

Creativity is what calisthenics is all about. Compared to lifting weights, you will have a lot more fun with calisthenics. Lifting weights is not bad per se. it helps achieve muscle growth and strength but there is also the tendency of getting tighter. On the contrary, calisthenics helps you attain flexibility, healthy joints, and you get to be in tune with your body. Furthermore, you get to work out in the environment of your choice. If you love being around nature outdoors, then you have it. It is like therapy. Some people have attested to healing injuries they have been dealing with for years by just doing calisthenics.

There are many myths based on calisthenics and one of them is that you cannot build muscle mass by doing calisthenics. This may have originated from gym enthusiasts who believe in weight lifting to gain mass. The sad part is that most of them have not tried one bit of calisthenics exercise. The truth of the matter is that, with calisthenics, your body is the weight you work with. That is quite a load. There is no additional weight, which could increase the risk of you getting hurt. You are your own gym.

Whether it is push-ups, pull ups, squats, or whatever calisthenics exercise you are doing, you are supposed to start with small reps and sets before you progressive. It is hardly unlikely that you will get up one morning and proceed to do 50 sets of push-ups. It takes time to build on the strength and your resistance. With time the body gets to adapt and you improve on the number of sets and with that, you also get to see a lot of improvement on your body.

Calisthenics provides you with an all-natural way of attaining body strength and weight. By all-natural it means you will hardly experience any side effects or injuries now and in the future. You have the ground, your body, and gravity all at your disposal. The rest is up to you to modify and ensure that you do it correctly. There is no excuse why you shouldn't be working out. If it is time, you only need to set a small percentage of the 24 hours you have per day to do calisthenics. It can actually be a refreshing way to kick-start your day.

The body is one huge mass made up of small muscles. In order for the body to be completely fit and healthy, these small bits of muscles all have to be fit. They are pieces of a bigger ship. If one part is not working properly then the rest of the body can't be said to be fit. Calisthenics helps you achieve fitness for the whole body all in a day's workout. It makes the body complete. There is hardly a muscle that is spared.

Discipline, hard work, and a healthy diet all go hand in hand with a good calisthenics work out. You should be able to achieve whatever it is you seek when you undertake your exercises correctly. Quality comes first before quantity. You have to get it right first before you think about increasing the number of sets and reps in your routine.

Chapter 2. Exercises

exercises (calisthenics uses mainly bodyweight exercises), give examples of these exercises. The more the better(ten or more). give the exercise name, then say something about it.

Push-ups

This happens to be the most common calisthenics exercise. It is one you have probably been doing but had no idea that is part of a calisthenics exercise. Push-ups are performed with the face down on the floor or forward, and the feet and hands shoulder width apart. The body should be straight from your heel all the way to the head.

The arms are often used to lift the body. You start with lowering the chest by bending the elbows to 90^0. You are not to rest on the floor when in a low position. The exercise works on a strong chest, triceps and shoulders. There are several variations which include the fingertip push-ups and the triceps push-ups. With the fingertips pusher up, you will be using the fingertips to support the weight and it helps improve grip strength and works on forearms. The triceps push-ups positioning is in a way that the hands are placed together under the chest with the fingers spread.

Dips

This exercise is performed between parallel bars. You place your arms on the bars and feet stretched in front of you. The body is then supposed to be lowered to the extent that elbows and shoulders get to be in line. You are then supposed to push up until the arms are extended fully. This exercise works on your chest, triceps, deltoids, and shoulders.

Pull-ups

You grab an overhead horizontal bar with your arms shoulder-width apart. You then proceed to lift your body up to the point where the bar is at par with your chin. The back should remain straight throughout the reps. It helps work the arms and the back. You can change the grip variations to wide or narrow. With an underhand grip, it is known as chin-up exercise and helps work the back and the biceps.

Inclined pull-ups

These pull-ups on the other hand are conducted on a lower bar where you lie or sit on the deck with your chest under the bar. With the hands placed at shoulder width and palms out, you pull the upper body towards the bar at 45^0. It works the arms, back, and shoulders.

Squats

The feet and shoulders should be width apart. You are then required to squat as far low as possible with your arms forward parallel to the floor. You will then return to standing position. It helps to train the calves, gluteals, quadriceps, and hamstrings. Variations include the squat jumps, hack squats, one-legged squats, and the wall squats. The squat jump is performed in the same position as the squats only that you will have to include a plyometric jumping movement whereby you are to jump as high as possible. The wall squats are done against a wall. With this exercise, you are required to conduct static holds where you pause every ¼ way of the movement and count 30 seconds before proceeding. With time you will increase the time as you grow stronger.

Lunges

This is performed by putting bringing one leg forward and lowering it till it forms a 90^0 angle and the back leg knee almost touching the ground. You are then supposed to stand up and alternate the legs. The back has to be straight and chest out. Variations of lunges include alternating lunges, non alternating lunges, side lunges, and crossover lunges. The alternating and non alternating lunges are done with either the front or the back leg elevated. The crossover lunges on the other hand are performed while one lunges to the side instead of forward. They all help to improve strength of the leg and stability.

Sit ups

It is performed by lying down on the floor with your back. Wrap your hands behind your head. The knees should be bent and you are required to raise your upper body off the floor and bring your chest closer to your knees. You then lower the back slowly to the floor which is the starting position and repeat the procedure. This exercise works on your abdominal muscles.

Crunches

This is almost similar to the sit ups only that while lying on your back, your knees have to be bent at 90^0. In this case, you will not be required to raise your whole torso area. You will perform short concentrated movements of the abdominals. It helps to work abdominals and obliques.

Calf raises

Stand on a raised platform with an edge with your heels hanging. Lift your entire body with your feet and then return to starting position. It helps to train the calf muscles. The different variations will be performed with toes pointed inward, turned outward, and straight forward.

Prone back extension

You lie with your face down and hands folded behind your head. You are then supposed to lift your upper torso until the chest and shoulders and off the ground. Hold that position for 3-5 seconds after which you return to the start position. It helps work the lower back. The variations include placing the hands behind the back or straight forward.

Leg raises

Lie on your back then raise your legs and move them up and down in slow movements. The hands can be placed under your buttocks or behind your head. The exercise puts strain on the abdominal muscles thus working them out effectively.

Plank

This exercise involves holding the top position of a push up for an extended period. It helps work on the rectus abdominis muscle.

Superman

Lie on your stomach and lift an opposite arm and leg 6 inches off the ground. Hold the position for 3-5 seconds. Lower the arm and leg then raise the opposite set. This helps to work on lower back and gluteals. To increase difficulty in variations, you can add weights to arms and legs.

Jumping jacks /stride jumps /star jumps

It is usually executed by jumping with legs spread wide and hands touching above your head. You then return to starting position with feet together and hands by your side. This is considered to be a full body work out. You can modify it in such a way that when returning to starting position, you assume a squatting position instead of standing so as to target the thigh, calf, gluteal, and abdominal muscles.

Chapter 3. Planning The Ideal Calisthenics Workout Timetable

For your workout to be effective and to get the results of its maximum level, you need to put in place a routine that has to be followed religiously. You will need a time span after which you can progress to more intense exercises once you are have succeeded in completing the first one. This timetable will include the number of sets and reps to be conducted during each work out and the number of weeks which you will be exercising. That is because you will need to have rest days to let the muscles to develop.

The workouts that you draw up in your timetable should be able to cover up most of the body muscles exercise. These include the legs, the chest, arms, and the abs. all these areas are very important. You should keep all of them in mind while drawing your time table. A timetable that involves you working out the entire week wouldn't be a good idea since the muscles have to be given some days off. Working out three or four days a week gives you room to carry out other body exercises such as cardio and resting too. Your daily schedule such as work engagements also have to be considered.

Three days per week starting with Monday then Wednesday and finally Friday would be ideal. This is because it is evenly spaced out during the week. It gives one time to prepare psychologically and physically for the next work out. Calisthenics is not a one day thing that one gets to achieve results overnight. It takes time which would require patience and determination. Most people often give up after a couple of days' workout and they do not see results. It could be they were not patient enough or more importantly, they were not doing the exercises the right way. Doing it right is one of the sole reasons why you should have a timetable.

To better understand how to draw up your timetable, let us look at the body muscles briefly and the exercises that can be used to work on them:

The chest

In working up the chest, the best exercises would be push-ups and chest dip. For the push ups there are other variations such as the one hand push up, inclined push up, and decline push up. In all the cases, the first step is to get it right. Once you have achieved that, you can then proceed to deal with increasing the rep ranges. Later on you can proceed to add weight whereby you could have someone stand near you and push down on your back. With the chest dip, you only have to ensure that you are safe. Setting the apparatus wrongly could easily lead to injury.

Back

Here you will have the chin ups and the under hand chin ups. Both exercises can be used to build a strong and nice back. The difference between the two is the grip. The underhand grip is always more comfortable because you will be able to lift more. Just like with the chest exercises, you have to work through the reps as your progress. Once you achieve high number of reps you can use some bit of resistance.

Hypertension can also be used for strengthening the lower back. However, you will need to have somebody standing nearby to watch over you or hold your feet to ensure you do not fall.

Thighs

Squats, lunges, glute-ham raise, and the straight-leg deadlift are all exercises that can be used to work out the thighs perfectly. They all help develop the quadriceps with a slight exception of the glute-ham raise which takes care of the hamstring.

Biceps and Triceps

Exercises for these two go hand in hand with those that are used for developing the chest and back. Therefore, while working on your chest and back, you will be taking care of more than just one muscle on your body. Pay attention to the curling of the biceps and triceps. Curling will mostly affect the bicep, uncurling the triceps. Doing each stage of these slowly in your workout will help you max out faster.

Abdominals and calf

These two will be developed by crunches and calf raises respectively.

Workout Routine For Monday, Wednesday and Friday

Push-ups   —   3 sets, maximum reps

Chin ups   —   3 sets, maximum reps

Hypertension -   2 sets, maximum reps

Squats   -   3 sets, maximum reps

Single leg squats-   3 sets, 4 maximum reps

Lunges   -   4 sets while alternating
the front and back legs

Bench dips   -   3 sets, maximum reps

Calf raises   -   3 sets, maximum reps

Ham-glute raises -   3 sets, maximum reps

Upside down shoulder press 3 sets, maximum reps

Sit ups   -   4 sets, maximum reps

Crunches   -   5 sets, 25 reps

Neck   -   3 sets, maximum reps

The duration you will be exercising during one workout session will depend on how well you execute the sets and how fast you complete the reps. However, it is advisable not to rush anything especially if you are just starting out on your routine. The most important thing is to do it properly.

About Your Workout Day

Planning your calisthenics work out day should pay attention to your current body strength, your availability and your goals. Moreover, you should factor in your environment to ensure that you make use of time in the most effective way possible.

Knowing your environment, for instance, will help factor in locations when planning your workout day. If you have to get to the park or rooftop to access some bars, you could opt to run or do the stairs other than taking the bus or lift. In this way, you will need less time to attain your goal and will end up working out more.

Just like regular gym workout schedules, calisthenics schedules should give your muscles time to recover and grow. Not all days should be hard out, full of excruciating exercise. Take a schedule that alternates between hard-core workout routines with soft sessions that will keep you moving without pushing you to the limit. This will give you motivation to face the next day whilst leaving you strong enough to carry on with your daily life.

When mixing up the proposed exercises, ensure that you do a balanced out choice. Choose something for your leg muscles, your abdomen and your upper body. Ensuring that these workout are vigorous enough should complement the cardio exercise you take. An all-round approach to your workout will ensure that you grow your body proportionally. This could be the difference between gym strength and calisthenics strength. With calisthenics, you are evenly strong. You can pull yourself over walls, or go up a flight of stairs carrying heavy grocery. You will attain true fitness and versatility that will help you in daily life.

Chapter 4. Additional Tips

The body is a system

Most regular gym exercise target specific body parts. Bench press for your chest and upper arms. Curls for your biceps. Squats for your rear. This is a good way to optimizing exercise. The only problem is that it could tempt you to underutilizing some parts of your body. The result is a poorly built up body rather than a properly proportioned layout.

With calisthenics, the body is a complete system that can never be split into parts. Using your entire body in working out ensures a proper cohesion of all your muscles. Unless you are working out for looks and not strength, you can never make it with specific workout.

The abs and calisthenics

Gaining abs with calisthenics is very simple. This is so since the abs form the core of every exercise you do. Everything you do with your body. This means if you go through all your exercise schedule properly, you will not have to invest in tummy trimmers or weighted sit ups to bring out your abs. However, if you must, you have to try the calisthenics workout aspect.

The exercise bar would be the right place to start from. You have to note that calisthenics abs are highly natural and good looking. To achieve them, you could use the leg raises at the exercise bar or windshield wipers. To the beginner, these exercises will max you very fast. Their results will be impressive.

Investing in an exercise bar

Most upper body and abdomen calisthenics depend on the exercise bar. While you might not have the exercise bar in your garage or neighborhood, investing in a safe one will ensure that you get your exercise right at all times. For instance, you could decide to choose a strong metallic water pipe installed in your basement. You could work with the swing crossbar at the park or decide to go with an overhanging branch from a tree in your yard.

Either way, you will need a strong surface you can grab with your hands. Something that can support one and half times your weight without bowing or breaking. If you do not intent to convert your calisthenics sessions into gymnastics, this improvising will be good enough. You will have a surface you can use to run your exercises safely and the clearance you need to attain an effective body.

Safety first

Some calisthenics are extreme. Calisthenics is like gymnastics or martial arts. You have to be a master before you can try some things. If you are to work out on your own, limit attempts to new and complex moves to safe areas. For instance, do not do inverted push-ups alone. Elevated push-ups require you to lift your legs up and balance on your arms. If you have not perfected the art, you can drop onto your chin harming yourself. If you must try this, have someone nearby, preferably an expert.

Other than exercising caution when trying out new procedures, you should also ensure that the props and surfaces you use to workout are safe and secure. Constantly check your exercise bars to ensure that they are firmly fixed before using them. Ensure that the floor is clean of any sharp objects before dropping down to do some push-ups or sit ups. This will go a long way into ensuring that you stay safe during the entire workout session.

Conclusion

Staying fit by working hard is crucial. Even though many people prefer doing this by visiting the gym, working out in the open will make it more practical and effective. With a regular and effective calisthenics schedule, you will not only work on boosting your cardio but also ensure that you work out every muscle in your body. The key to proper calisthenics lies in understanding your muscles and constantly adding on exercise schedules that will target different parts of your body.

Regardless of how good your schedule is, you will need dedication to survive. Setting aside some ample time of the day for your workout is the best way out. Some people prefer working out in the evening after work before resting. Others prefer doing it in the day. If you work during the day, morning workouts might leave you tired especially if they are rigorous. Choosing what will perfectly fit into your schedule is the ultimate way to choosing the right exercise time. After this, all you will need is the perfect calisthenics routine and you are good to go.

Thank You Page

I want to personally thank you for reading my book. I hope you found information in this book useful and I would be very grateful if you could leave your honest review about this book. I certainly want to thank you in advance for doing this.

If you have the time, you can check my other books too.

Lightning Source UK Ltd.
Milton Keynes UK
UKHW021313121122
412097UK00018B/177